Careers without College

Nurse Assistant

by Kathryn A. Quinlan

Consultants:

Sandra Cochran, RN, BS, MAM
Director of Nurses, Program Director CNA/CHHA
California Paramedical and Technical College

Diana Dugan, RN
Nursing Assistant Instructor
Pima Medical Institute
Tucson, Arizona

CAPSTONE
HIGH/LOW BOOKS
an imprint of Capstone Press
Mankato, Minnesota

Capstone High/Low Books are published by Capstone Press
818 North Willow Street • Mankato, MN 56001
http://www.capstone-press.com

Copyright © 1999 Capstone Press. All rights reserved.
No part of this book may be reproduced without written permission from the publisher. The publisher takes no responsibility for the use of any of the materials or methods described in this book, nor for the products thereof.
Printed in the United States of America.

Library of Congress Cataloging-in-Publication Data
Quinlan, Kathryn A.
  Nurse assistant/by Kathryn A. Quinlan.
    p. cm. — (Careers without college)
  Includes bibliographical references and index.
  Summary: Outlines job responsibilities and the work environment of nurse assistants as well as the necessary training, job outlook, salary, and career potential.
  ISBN 0-7368-0036-0
  1. Nurses' aides—Vocational guidance—Juvenile literature. [1. Allied health personnel—Vocational guidance. 2. Vocational guidance.] I. Title. II. Series: Careers without college (Mankato, Minn.)
RT84.Q56 1999
610.73'06'98—DC21   98-17782
                                                                                  CIP
                                                                                   AC

Editorial Credits
Kimberly J. Graber, editor; James Franklin, cover designer/illustrator;
  Sheri Gosewisch, photo researcher
Photo Credits
Borland Stock Photo/Charlie Borland, 30
ColePhoto/Lee Snyder, 9; Mark Gibson, 14, 16, 24, 32
Impact Visuals/Jim West, 27, 39, 42
International Stock/Michael Parras, cover; Peter Krinninger, 12
PhotoBank, Inc./Grantpix, 6
Photo Network/Tom McCarthy, 4; Dennis McDonald, 34; Mike Moreland, 36
Shaffer Photography/James L. Shaffer, 19, 22
Unicorn Stock Photos/Tom McCarthy, 20, 29; Jeff Greenberg, 47
Visuals Unlimited/Jeff Greenberg, 11

Table of Contents

Fast Facts 5

Chapter 1   What Nurse Assistants Do 7

Chapter 2   What the Job Is Like 15

Chapter 3   Training 23

Chapter 4   Salary and Job Outlook 31

Chapter 5   Where the Job Can Lead 37

Words to Know 40

To Learn More 44

Useful Addresses 45

Internet Sites 46

Index 48

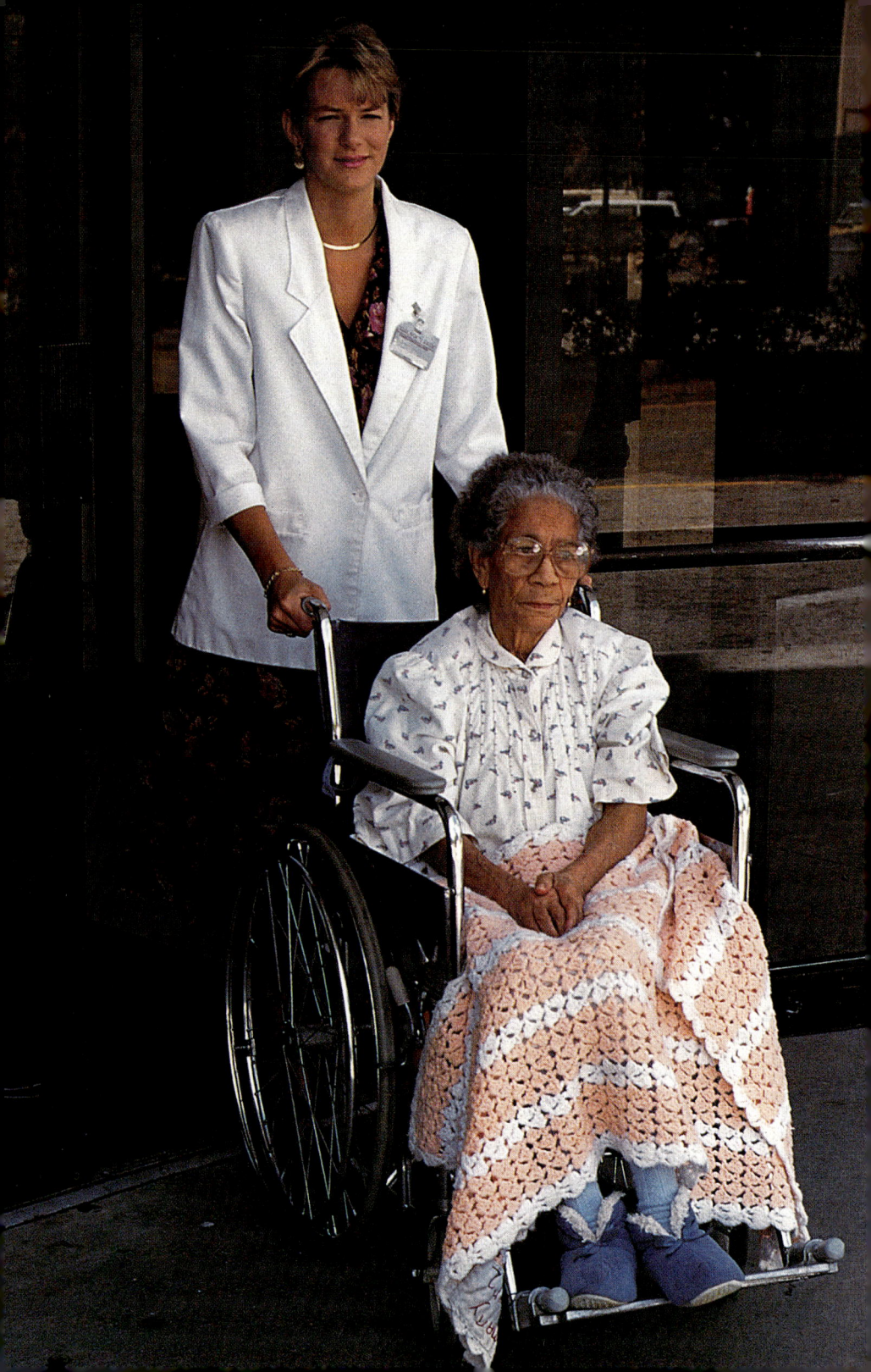

Fast Facts

Career Title _____ Nurse assistant

Minimum Educational _____ U.S.: some high school
Requirement and on-the-job training
Canada: some high school
and on-the-job training

Certification Requirement _____ U.S.: varies by state
Canada: none

Salary Range _____ U.S.: $9,828 to $26,364
(U.S. Bureau of Labor Statistics and
Human Resources Development Canada,
late 1990s figures) Canada: $9,000 to $36,900
(Canadian dollars)

Job Outlook _____ U.S.: faster than average growth
(U.S. Bureau of Labor Statistics and
Human Resources Development
Canada, late 1990s projections) Canada: stable

DOT Cluster _____ Service occupations
(Dictionary of Occupational Titles)

DOT Number _____ 355.674-014

GOE Number _____ 10.03.02
(Guide for Occupational Exploration)

NOC _____ 3413
(National Occupational Classification—Canada)

5

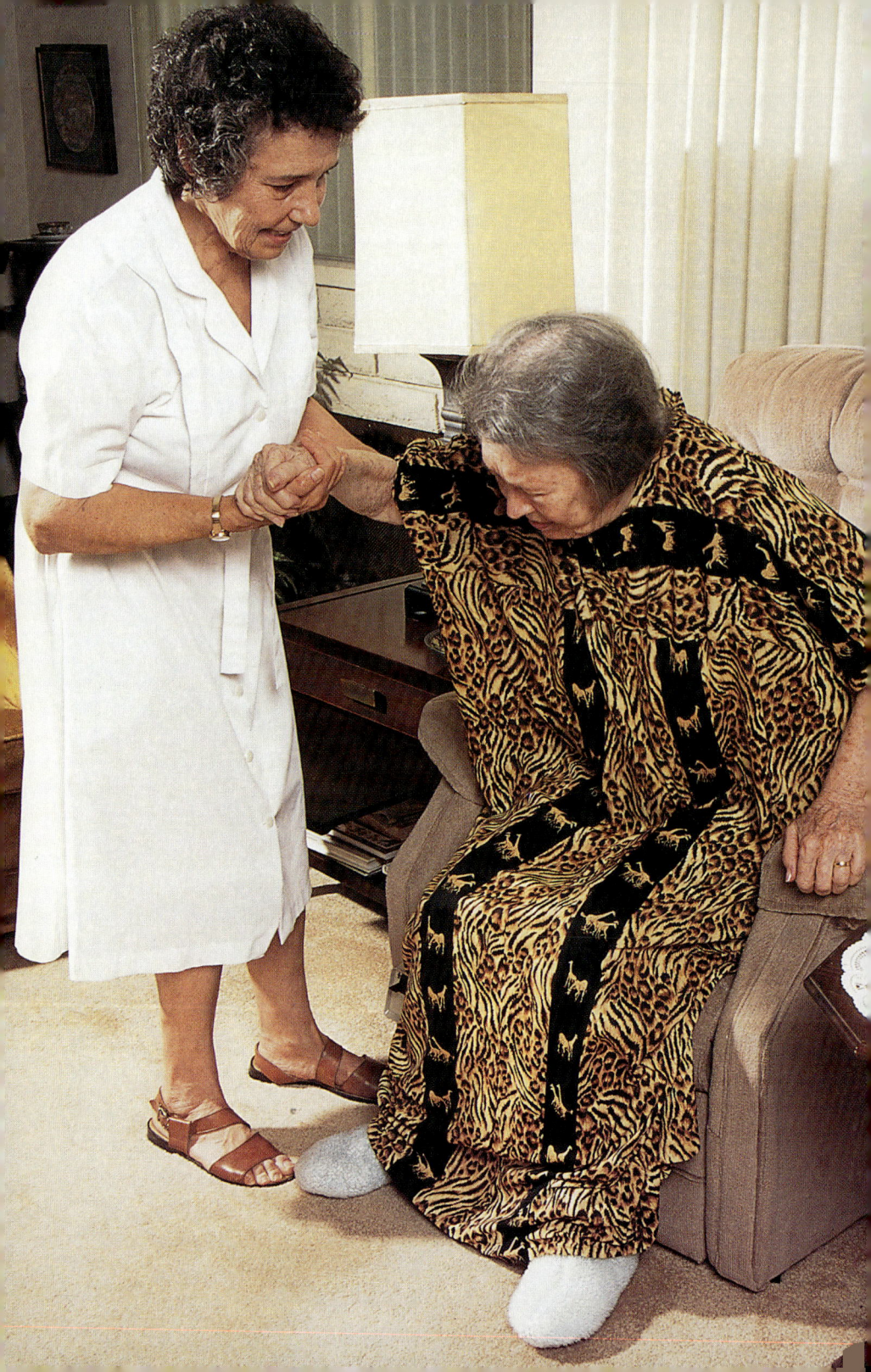

Chapter 1

What Nurse Assistants Do

Nurse assistants help doctors and nurses care for people who are sick, hurt, or disabled. People who are disabled have limited use of their bodies. Some people cannot walk. Some people cannot use their hands. Nurse assistants also care for older people. These nurse assistants are geriatric aides.

Nurse assistants care for older people.

On the Job

Nurse assistants help nurses by performing many common tasks. They clean rooms and order supplies. Nurse assistants make beds and serve meals.

Nurse assistants work closely with patients. Patients need help to eat, dress, and bathe. Nurse assistants answer patients' calls for assistance. They take patients to operating rooms and to examination rooms.

Medical Tests

Some nurse assistants perform basic medical tests. These nurse assistants have specialized training and experience. Nurse assistants check patients' body temperatures with thermometers. Healthy people have body temperatures of about 98.6 degrees Fahrenheit (37 degrees Celsius). A high body temperature can be a sign of illness.

Nurse assistants order supplies.

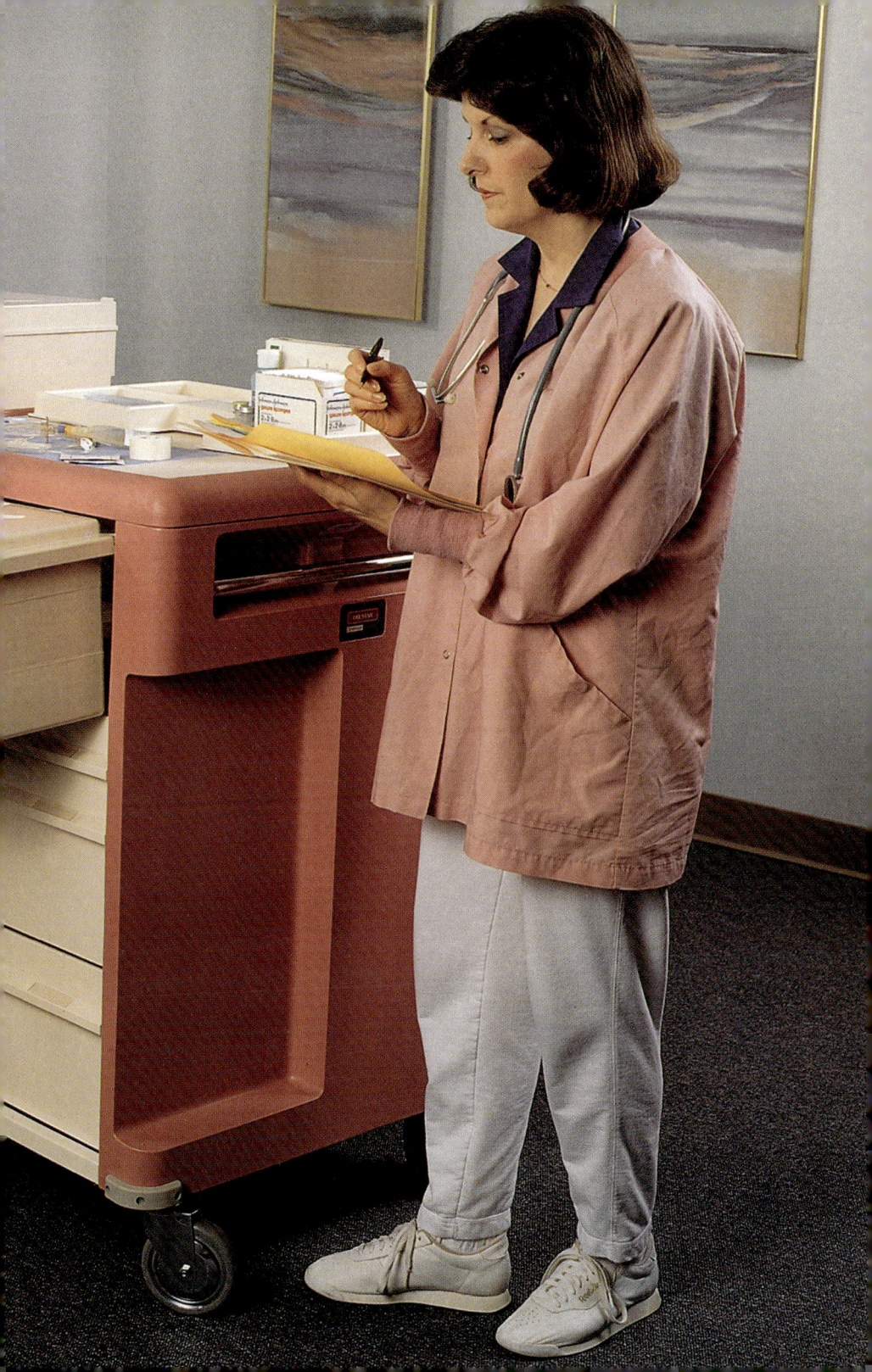

Nurse assistants check patients' pulses. This throbbing in the veins is caused by the heart as it pumps blood. Nurse assistants can feel a pulse by gently holding a patient's wrist. They also can feel it at several other points on the body. Nurse assistants count the number of beats per minute. A heart that beats too quickly or too slowly can signal a problem.

Nurse assistants check patients' breathing. They count the number of times patients breathe in one minute. Patients who breathe too quickly may have an illness of the lungs.

Nurse assistants check patients' blood pressure. Blood pressure is the force blood places on arteries as it moves through the body. High blood pressure can cause heart problems and other illnesses.

Nurse assistants write medical test results on patients' charts. Doctors and nurses check these charts as they care for patients. Nurse assistants tell doctors or nurses about unusual test results.

Nurse assistants record test results in patients' files.

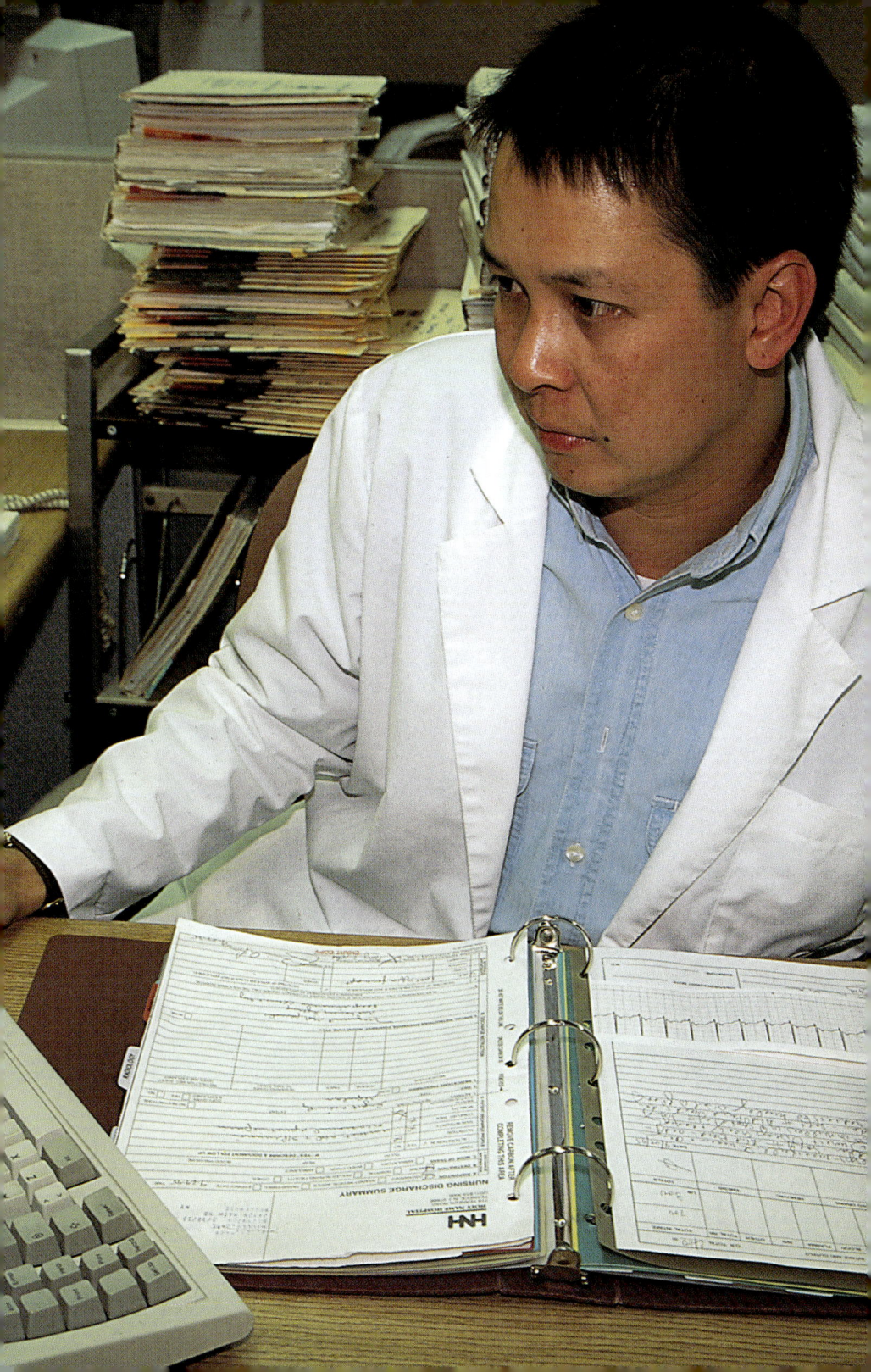

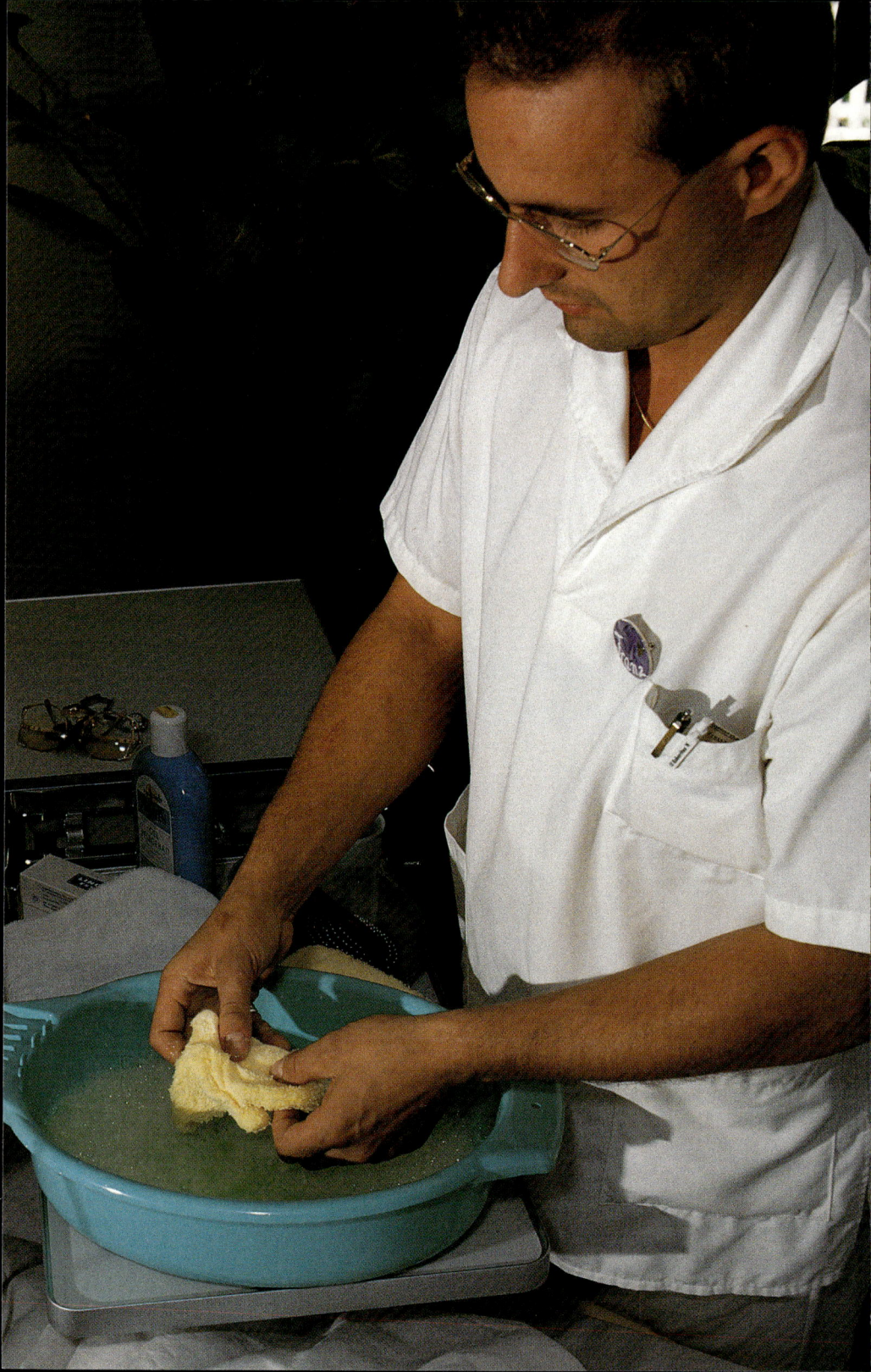

Working with Patients

Nurse assistants often have more contact with patients than other health care workers do. Nurse assistants may work with patients who are upset or in pain. Nurse assistants work to help patients relax. They try to cheer up patients by being friendly.

Nurse assistants help patients feel comfortable. They change dirty sheets. They also empty bedpans. Patients use bedpans when they need to use the bathroom but cannot get out of bed.

Nurse assistants help patients with activities that are usually private. These activities include bathing and dressing. Nurse assistants must be able to help patients without making them feel uncomfortable.

Many nurse assistants work in nursing homes. They may work with the same patients for many years. Nurse assistants often build friendships with these patients.

Nurse assistants help patients bathe.

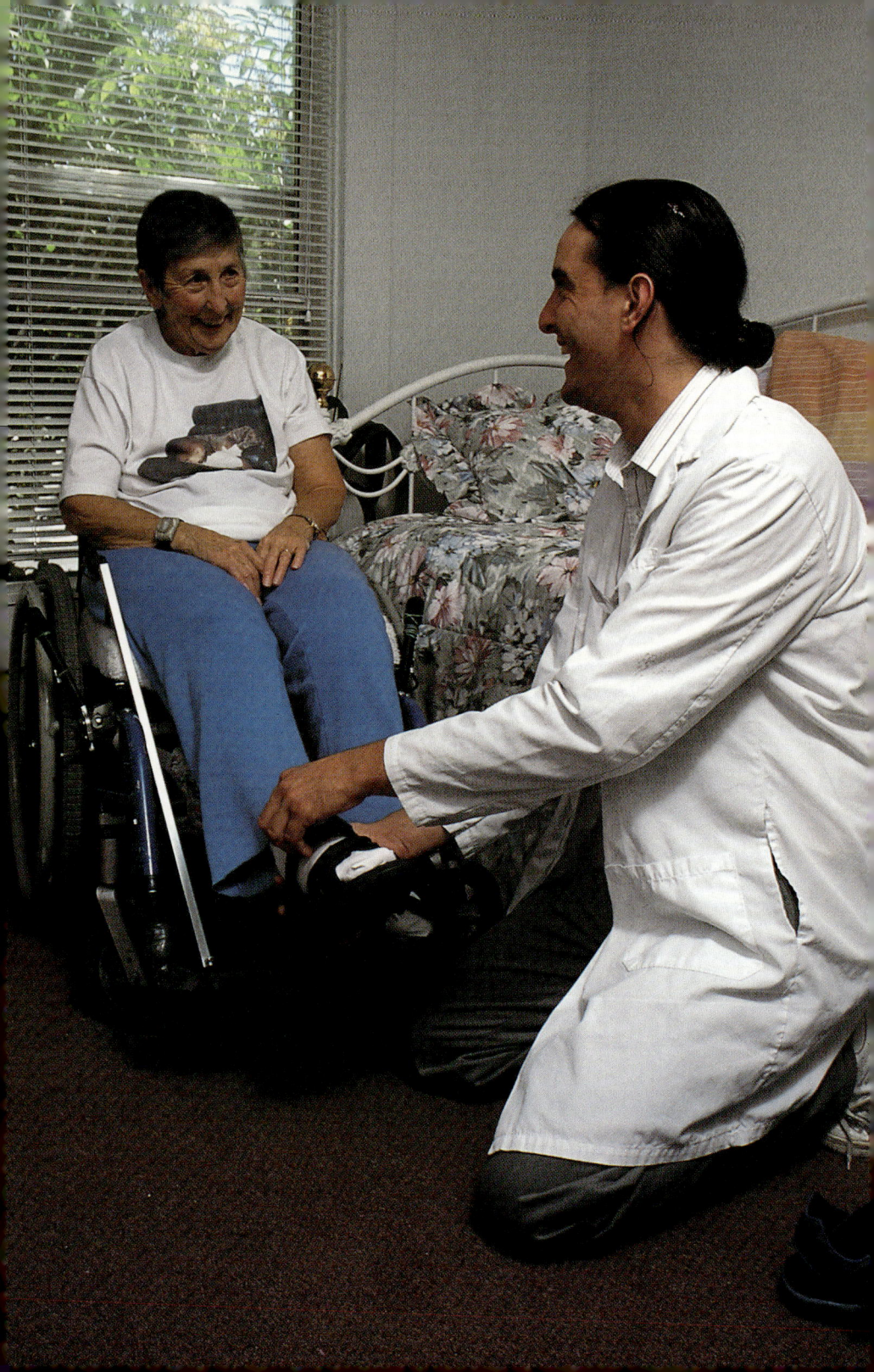

Chapter 2

What the Job Is Like

Nurse assistants work in many settings. They work in hospitals and nursing homes. Nurse assistants also provide care for older people and people with disabilities in residential care centers. People in these centers receive personal care and medical care if they need it. Some nurse assistants visit people in their homes. These nurse assistants are home health aides.

Some nurse assistants visit people in their homes.

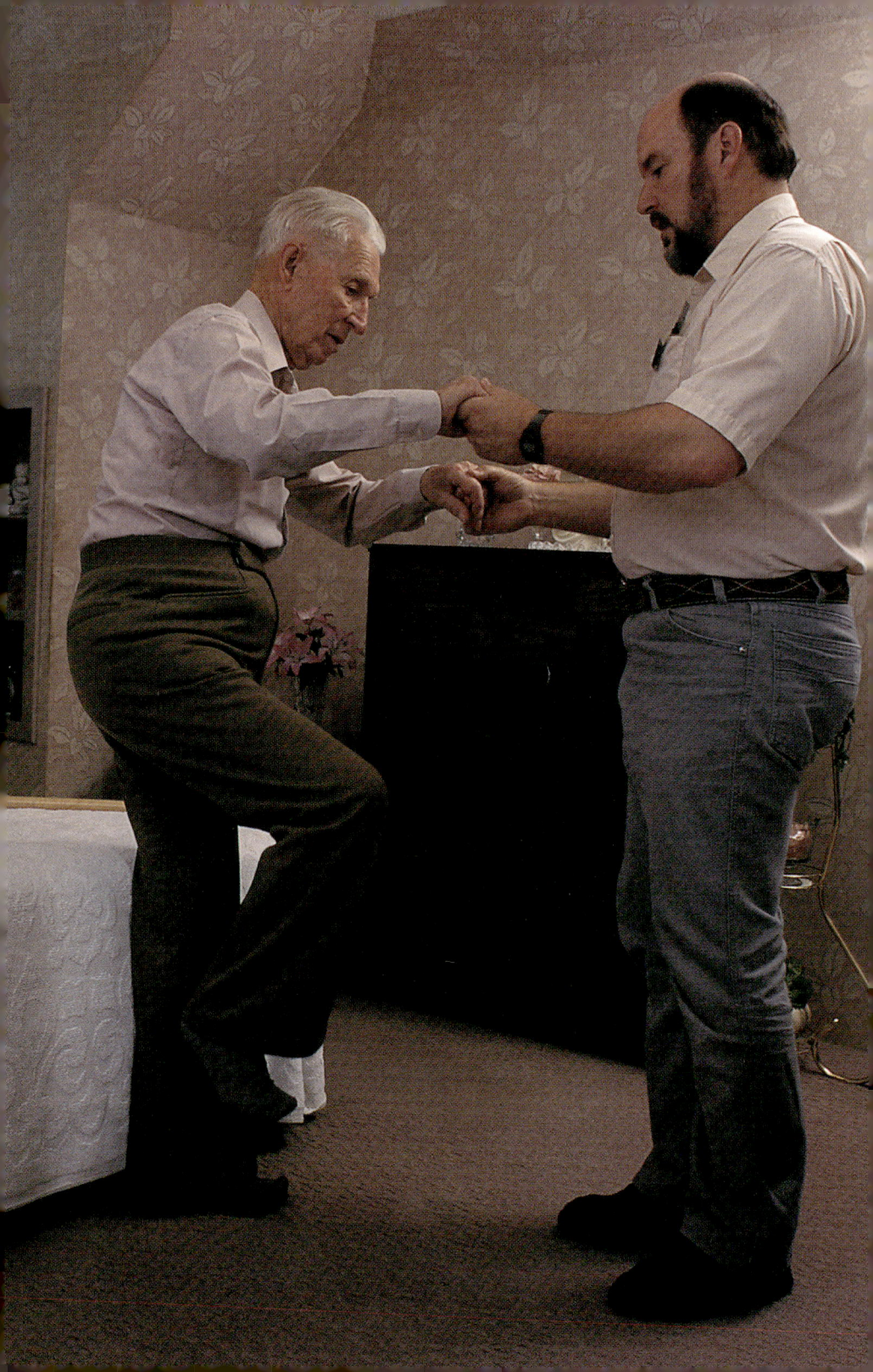

Nurse assistants' work hours vary depending on where they work. Many nurse assistants in hospitals and nursing homes work 40 hours per week. Some nurse assistants work part time. Part-time workers spend less than 40 hours per week at work. Many nurse assistants work nights and weekends. Some patients need care at all times.

Experienced nurse assistants often can choose the hours they work. Beginning nurse assistants usually must work nights, weekends, and holidays.

Work Environment

Nurse assistants work hard. They spend many hours on their feet. They move from room to room to check on patients. Nurse assistants help patients into and out of bed. They help patients stand, walk, and exercise.

Most nurse assistants care for several patients during each shift. Patients often have unexpected problems and need extra care. Nurse assistants must tend to these patients. Nurse assistants also must do all their regular tasks.

Nurse assistants help patients exercise.

17

Nurse assistants face challenges in their jobs. They sometimes work with patients who are unhappy or angry. They work with doctors and nurses who have pressure in their jobs. These co-workers can be demanding.

Nurse assistants face some risks. Nurse assistants can catch illnesses from patients. Nurse assistants also can hurt their backs if they lift patients incorrectly or without assistance. Most nurse assistants can stay healthy if they follow safety procedures.

Personal Qualities

Nurse assistants should be caring people. They should be polite, friendly, and cheerful. Patients often feel pain. Nurse assistants need to be calm and understanding. They should be good listeners. Patients often want to talk about their pain.

Nurse assistants must be able to communicate clearly and quickly. They should be able to alert doctors or nurses to problems. Nurse assistants

Nurse assistants should be friendly and cheerful.

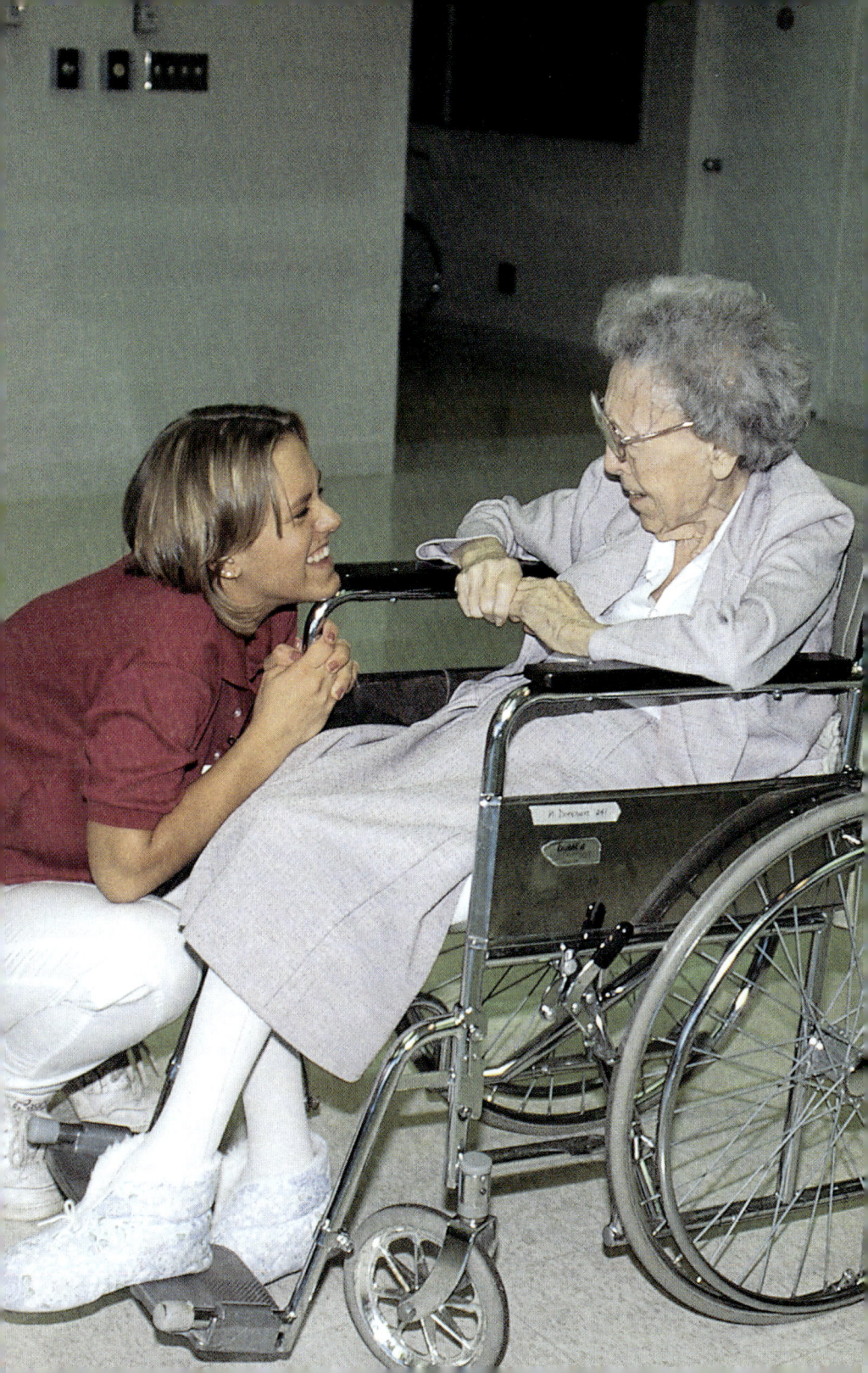

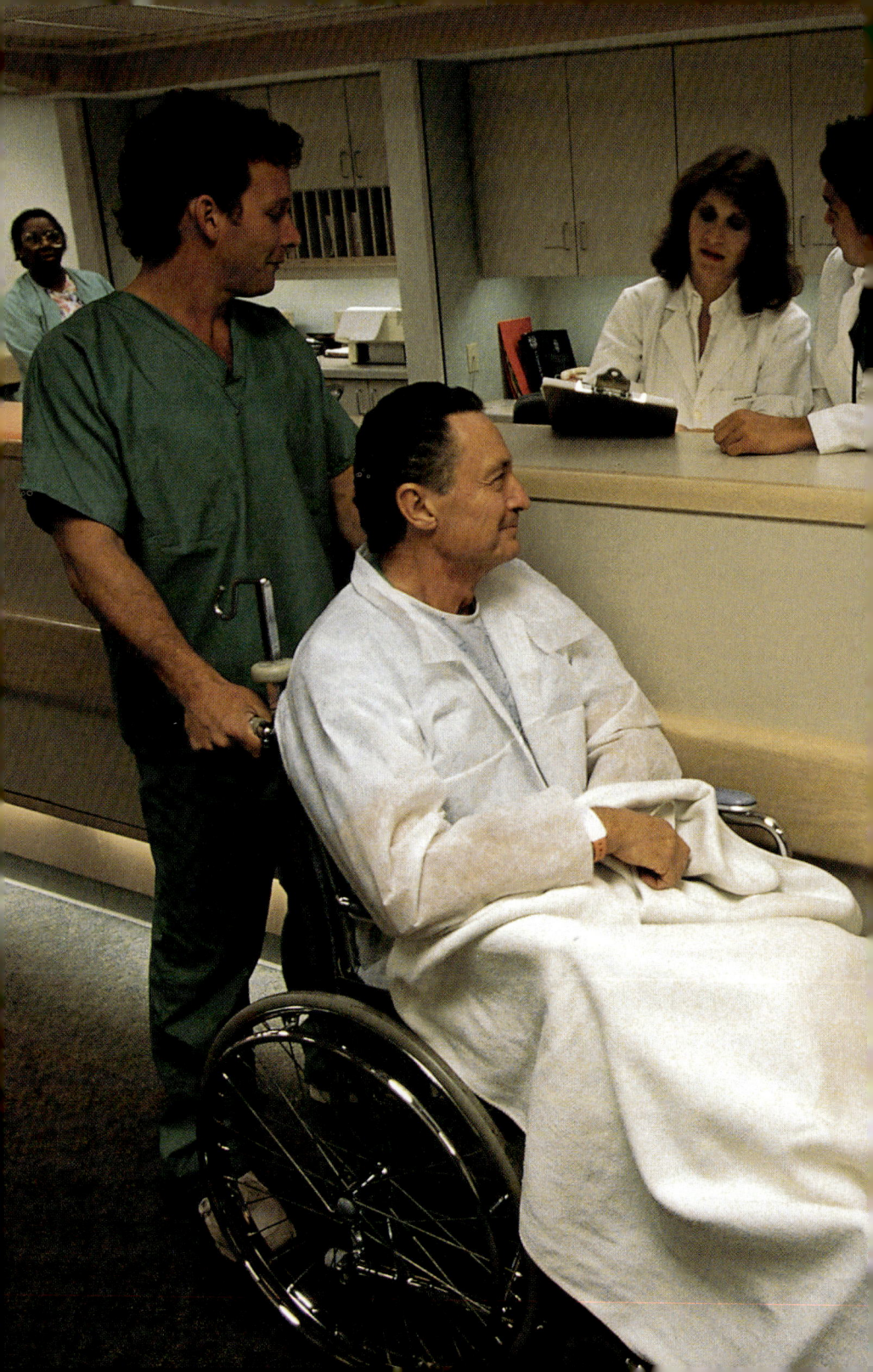

must work well in teams. Communication skills help them work well with other people.

Nurse assistants must be observant people. They need to be aware of small changes in patients. Nurse assistants should notice if patients seem uncomfortable or in pain.

Nurse assistants must be strong and fit. Many patients need help to stand and walk. Nurse assistants also must be able to push wheelchairs.

Most nurse assistants feel good about their work. They know they help people feel better. Nurse assistants also know nurses and doctors need their help to give patients good care.

Nurse assistants must be able to push wheelchairs.

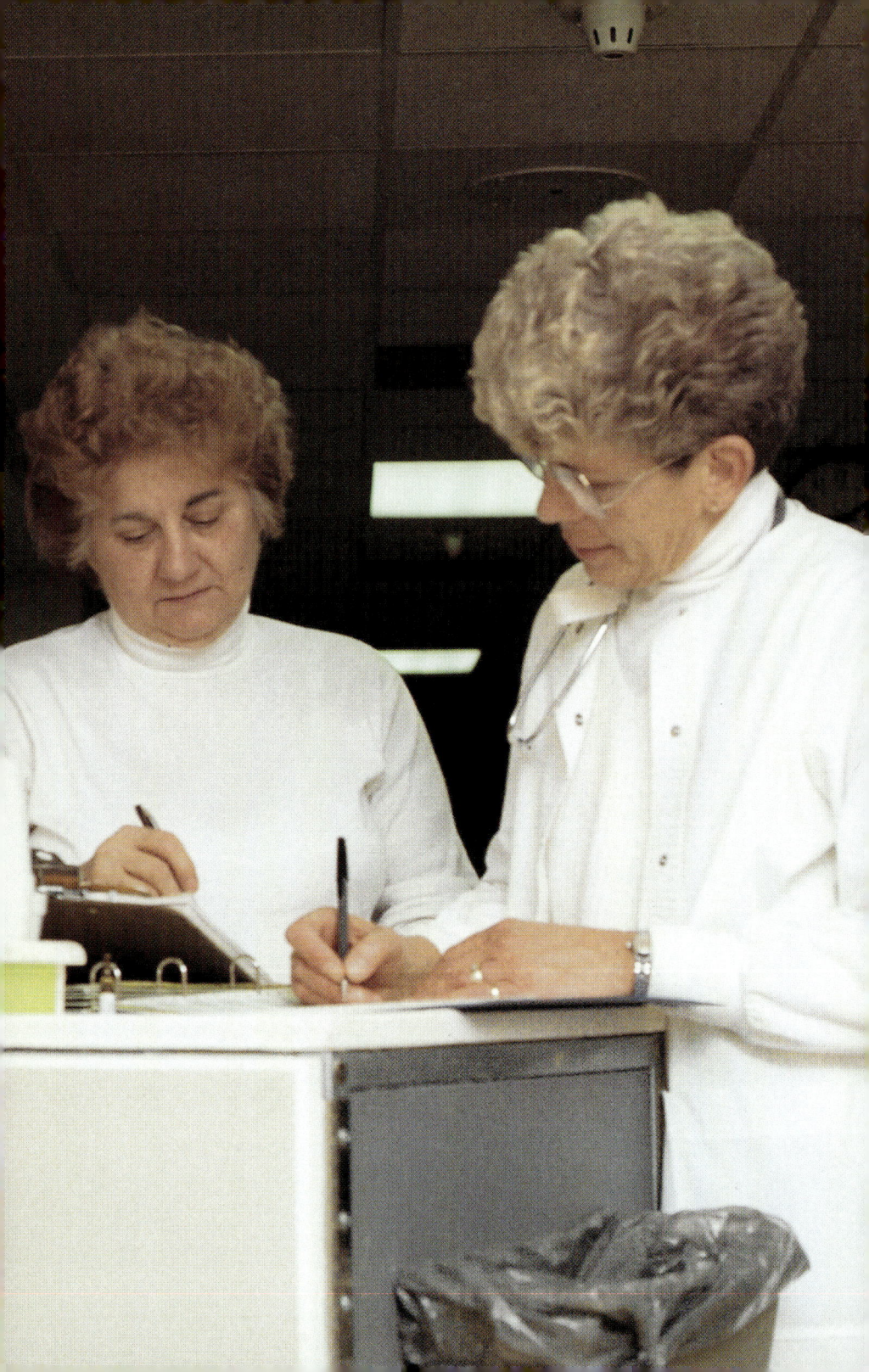

Chapter 3

Training

Nurse assistants have different levels of training. Many people enter the nurse assistant field after high school. Some nurse assistants enter the field before finishing high school. Most nurse assistants in the United States go through training programs at community colleges or vocational schools. These programs vary in length. They usually last a few months.

Schools in most areas of Canada offer nurse assistant training after high school. These programs last from a few months to nearly a year. High

Nurse assistants have different levels of training.

schools in Quebec offer nurse assistant training. Some areas of Canada require nurse assistants to have licenses.

Nurse assistant students study the human body in anatomy classes. Students learn about the science of nutrition. People who understand nutrition know how bodies use food to stay strong and healthy. Nurse assistant students also learn how to help patients bathe, dress, and eat.

Nurse assistants learn on the job. They work closely with experienced assistants and health care workers. Nurse assistants also may take classes at work, or they may attend classes outside of work. Each workplace has its own procedures.

Certified Nursing Assistants
In the United States, most nursing homes and many hospitals hire only certified nursing assistants (CNAs). Certified nursing assistants

Many hospitals hire only certified nursing assistants.

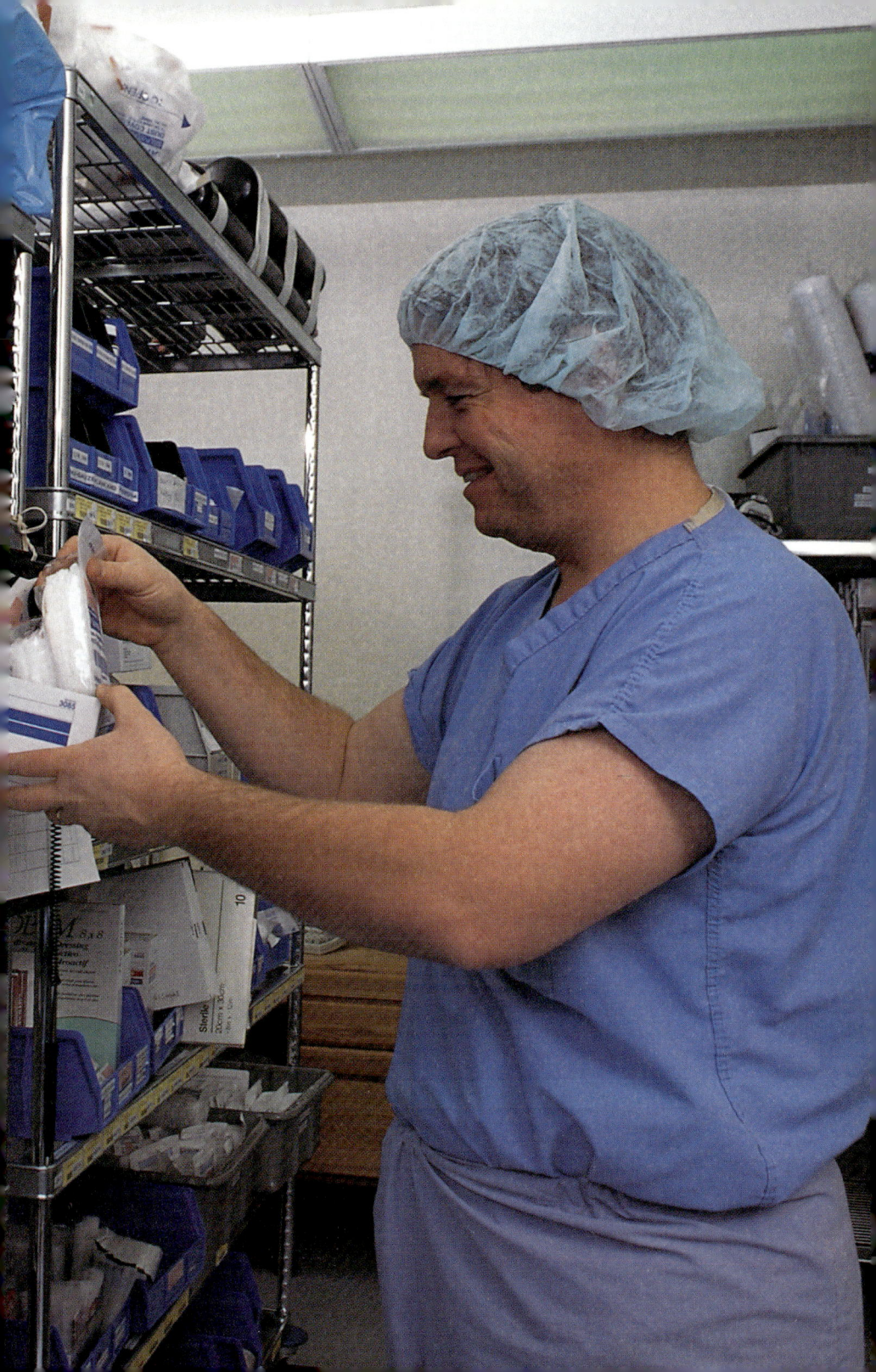

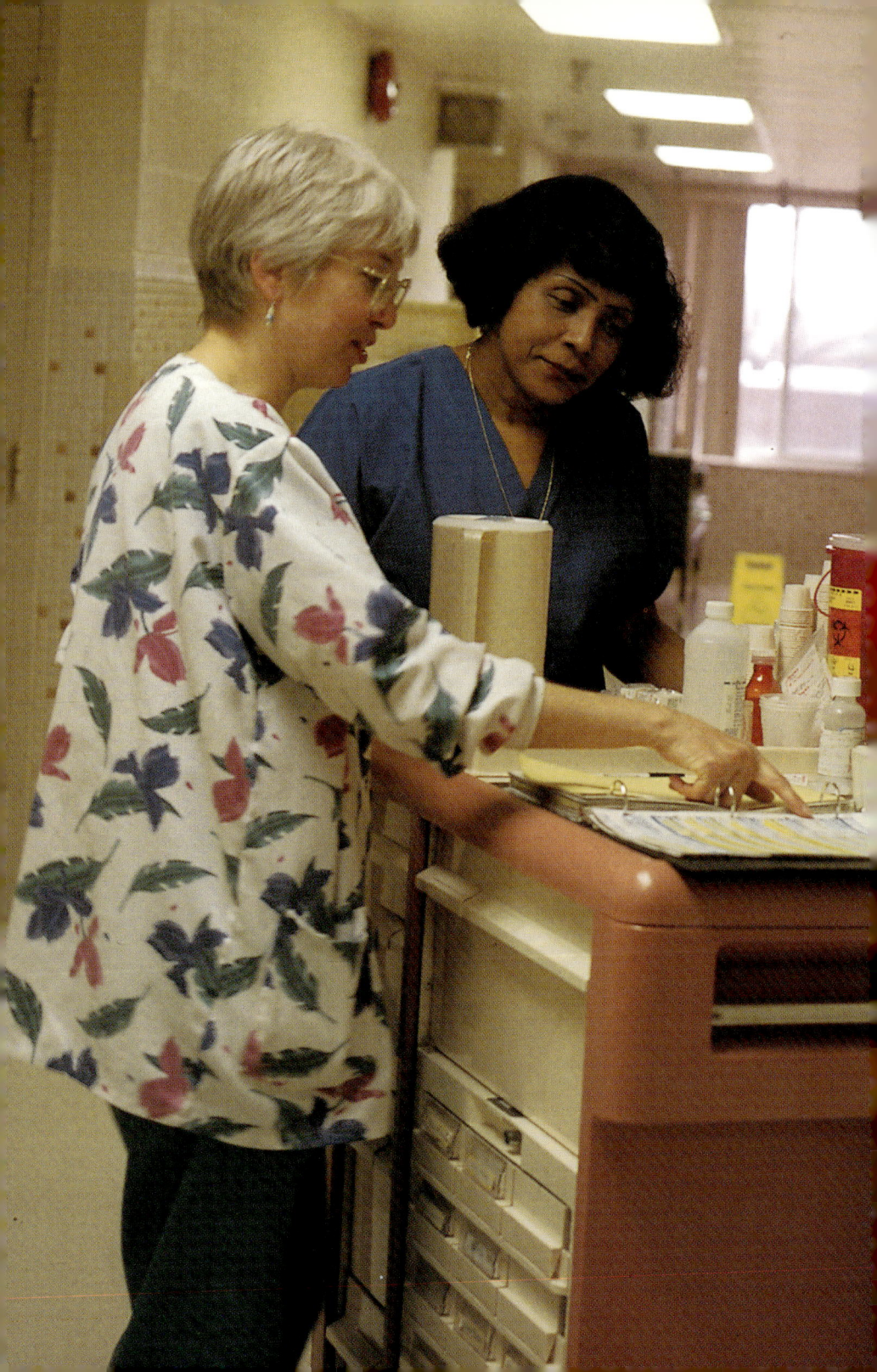

have officially recognized skills and abilities. Certified nursing assistants may find jobs more easily than those who are not certified.

People may decide to become CNAs at any time. Some people receive CNA training as soon as they begin working. Others may work as nurse assistants first. Even experienced nurse assistants must attend CNA training before they apply for certification.

Each state decides how much training CNAs must receive. Training may include class work and practical experience. People take written tests and skills tests to become CNAs.

CNAs may continue to take classes outside of work even after they are certified. This helps them learn new facts about patient care and health care work. CNAs may need to take additional classes to renew their certification. Requirements for renewal vary by state.

CNA training may include practical experience.

What Students Can Do Now

Students can volunteer in health care facilities if they want to be nurse assistants. Volunteers offer to do a job without pay. Nursing homes and hospitals often have jobs volunteers can do. Volunteers can learn hospital and nursing home procedures. They also can find out if they like working with patients.

High school students may be able to work as nurse assistants. Some health care facilities do not require nurse assistants to have high school diplomas. These nurse assistants often work after school and on weekends.

Students can volunteer in hospitals or nursing homes if they want to be nurse assistants.

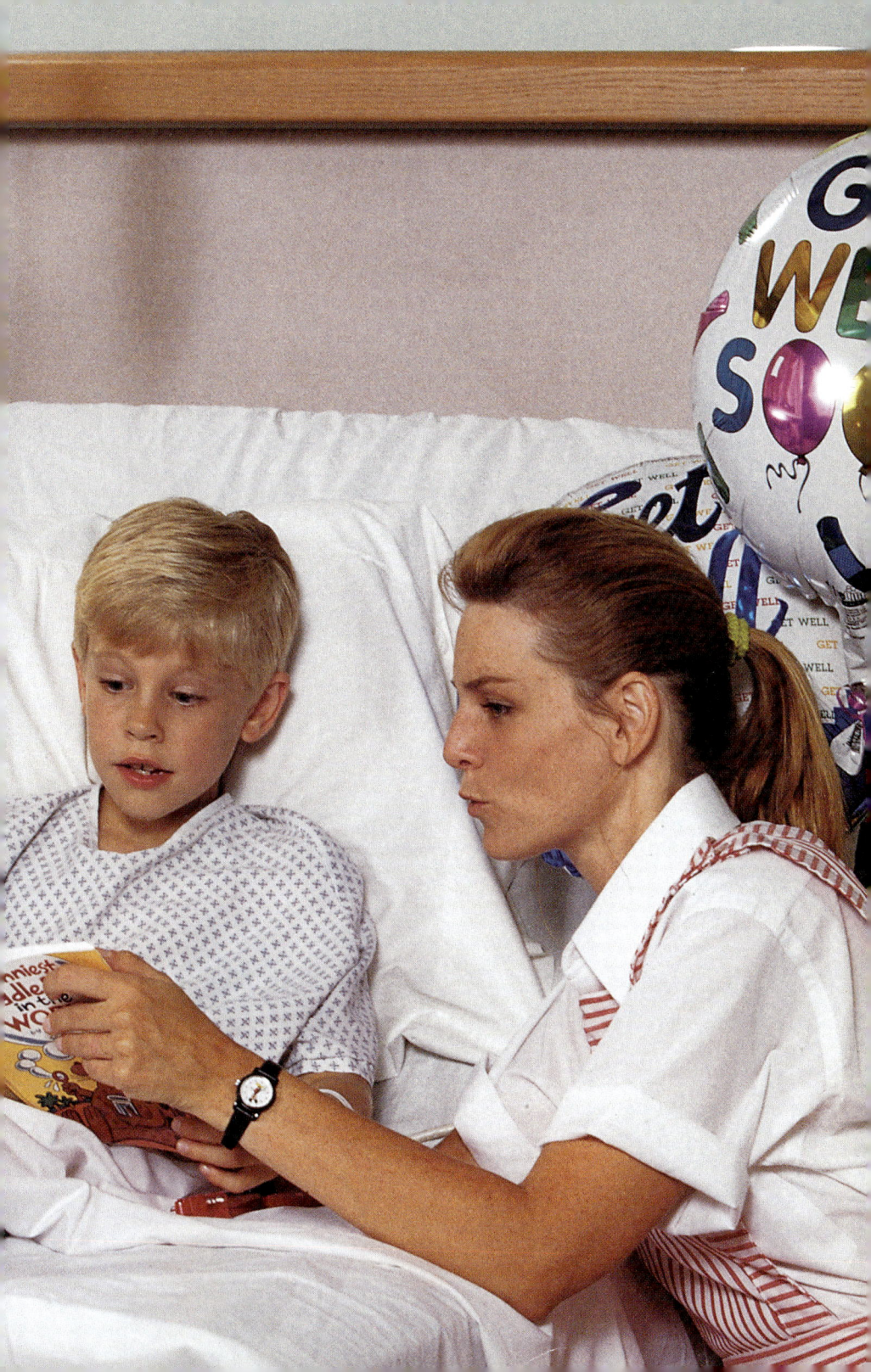

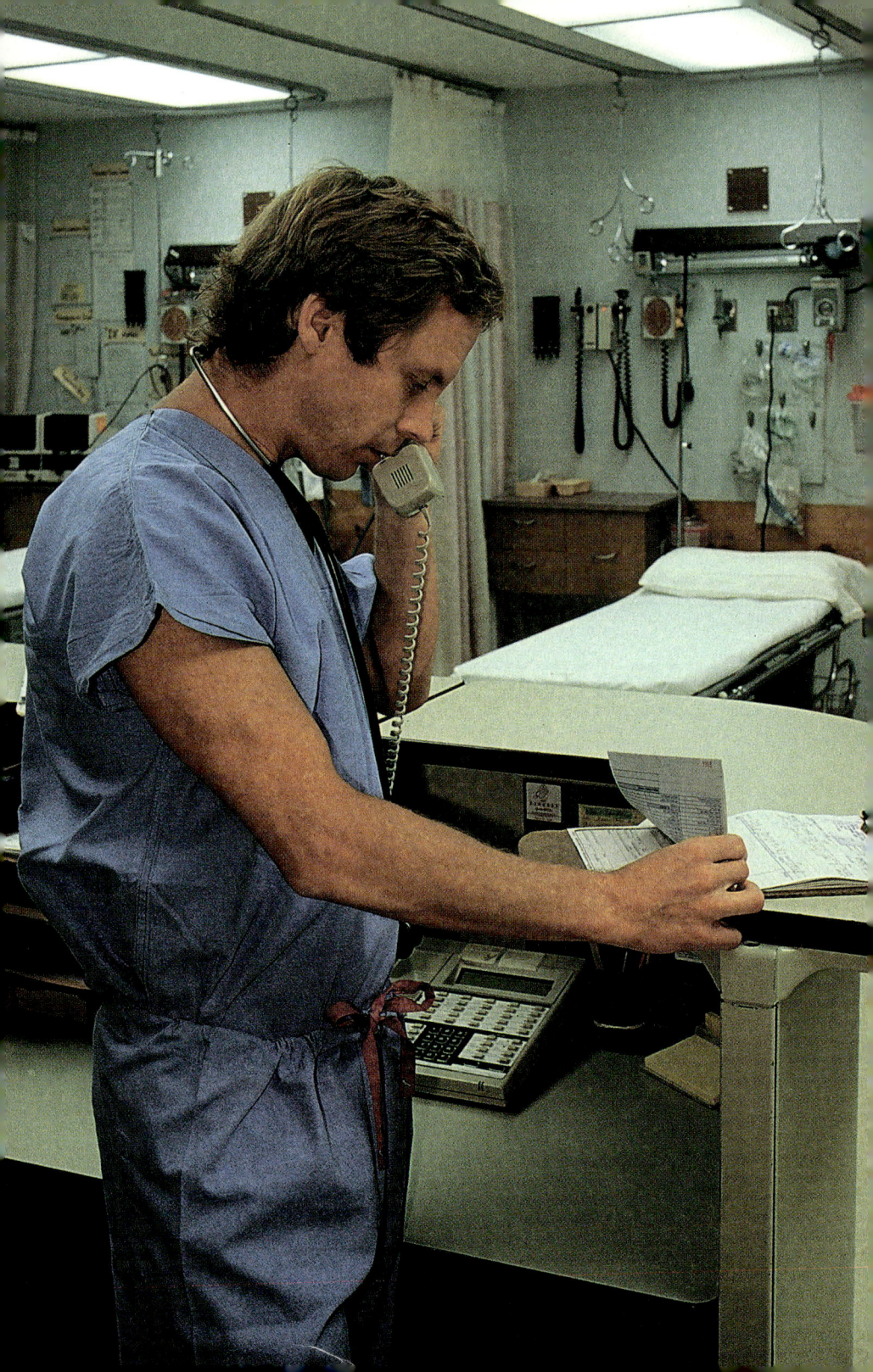

Chapter 4

Salary and Job Outlook

The amount of money nurse assistants earn depends on where they work. Nurse assistants who work in hospitals usually earn more than those who work in nursing homes. Large nursing homes and hospitals pay more than smaller facilities.

Nurse assistants who work in hospitals usually earn more than those who work in nursing homes.

Salary

Most nurse assistants in the United States earn between $12,100 and $19,300 per year (all figures late 1990s). The lowest amount full-time U.S. nurse assistants earn is about $9,800 per year. The highest amount assistants earn is about $26,400 per year.

The lowest amount full-time nurse assistants earn in Canada is about $9,000 per year. The highest amount they earn is about $36,900 per year. The average yearly salary for a nurse assistant in Canada is $21,700.

Job Outlook

The nurse assistant field is growing in the United States. It is growing for two reasons. First, people live longer than they did in the past. People have more health problems as they age. Nursing homes and residential care centers need more nurse assistants to care for these people.

People have more health problems as they age.

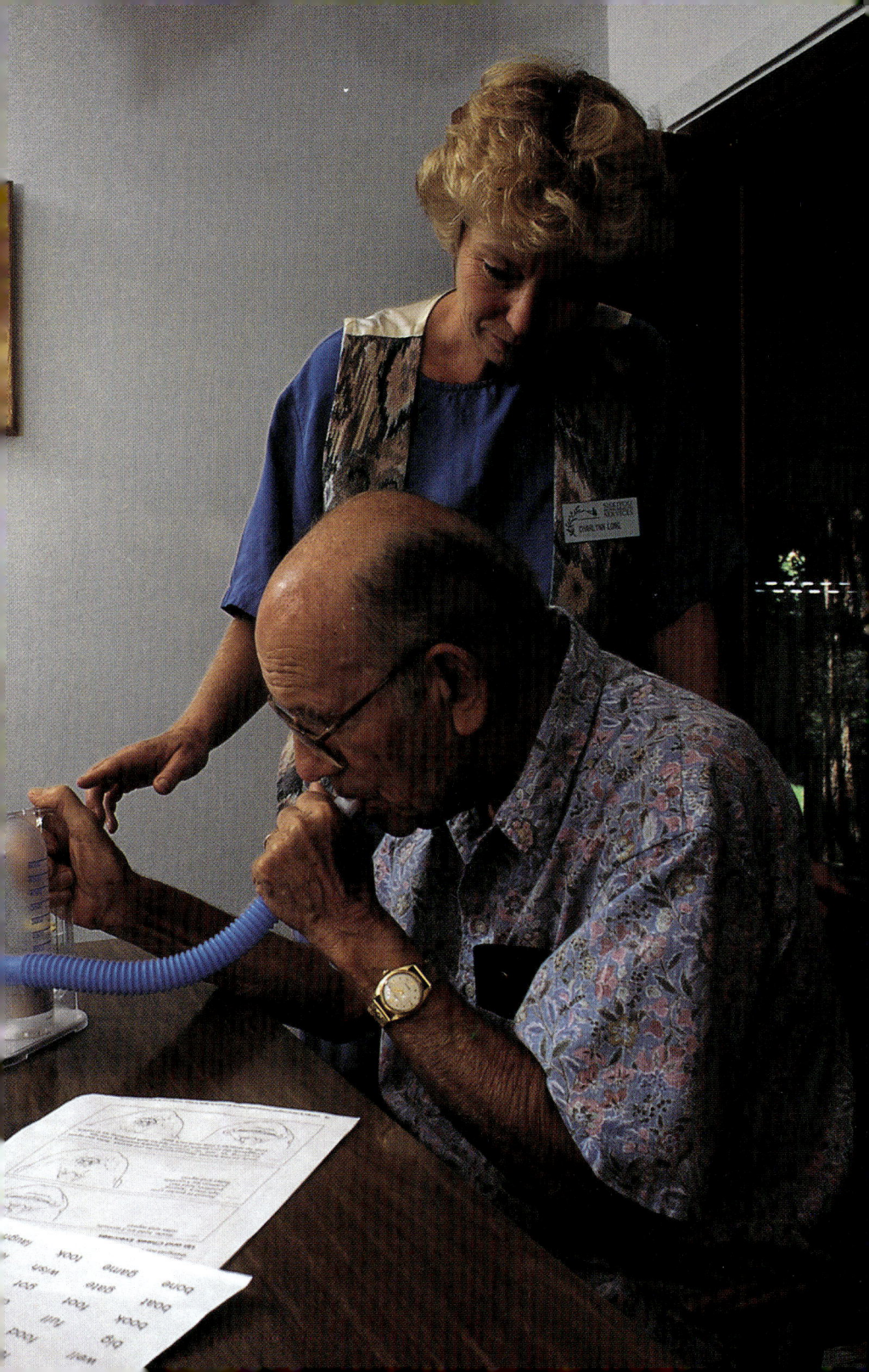

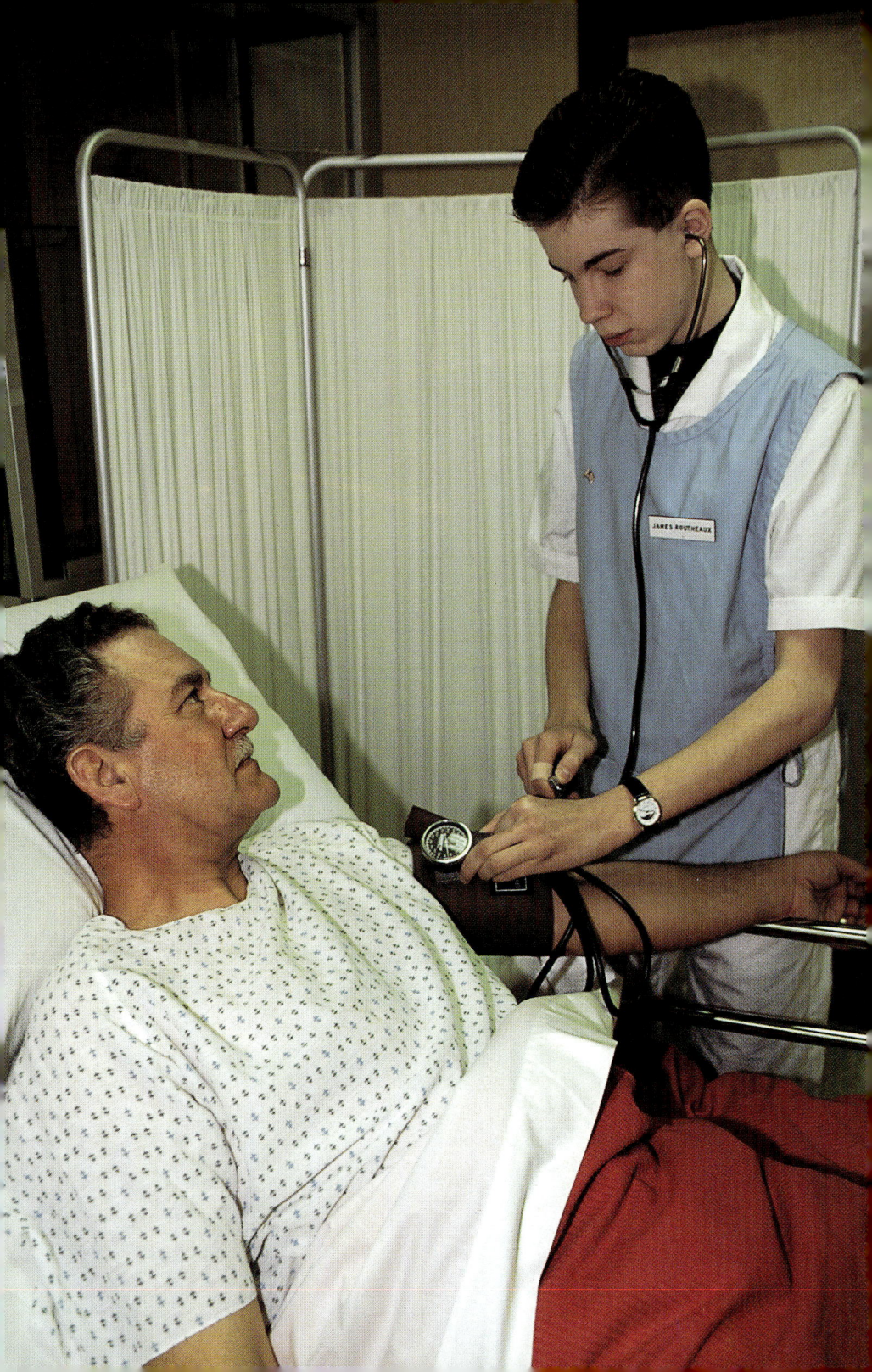

Second, hospitals try to keep the costs of providing health care as low as possible. Nurse assistants complete basic tasks. This allows doctors and nurses to treat more patients and perform more technical tasks. Hospitals can hire fewer nurses and doctors. Nurse assistants earn less than doctors or nurses. Nurse assistants help hospitals and nursing homes to care for more patients for less money.

The nurse assistant field is stable in Canada. The number of available jobs is staying about the same as in previous years. Hospitals are hiring fewer workers. But Canadians also are living longer than they did in the past. Older Canadians need help caring for themselves. Most nurse assistant jobs in Canada are in nursing homes and residential care centers.

Nurse assistants perform basic tasks. This allows doctors and nurses to treat more patients.

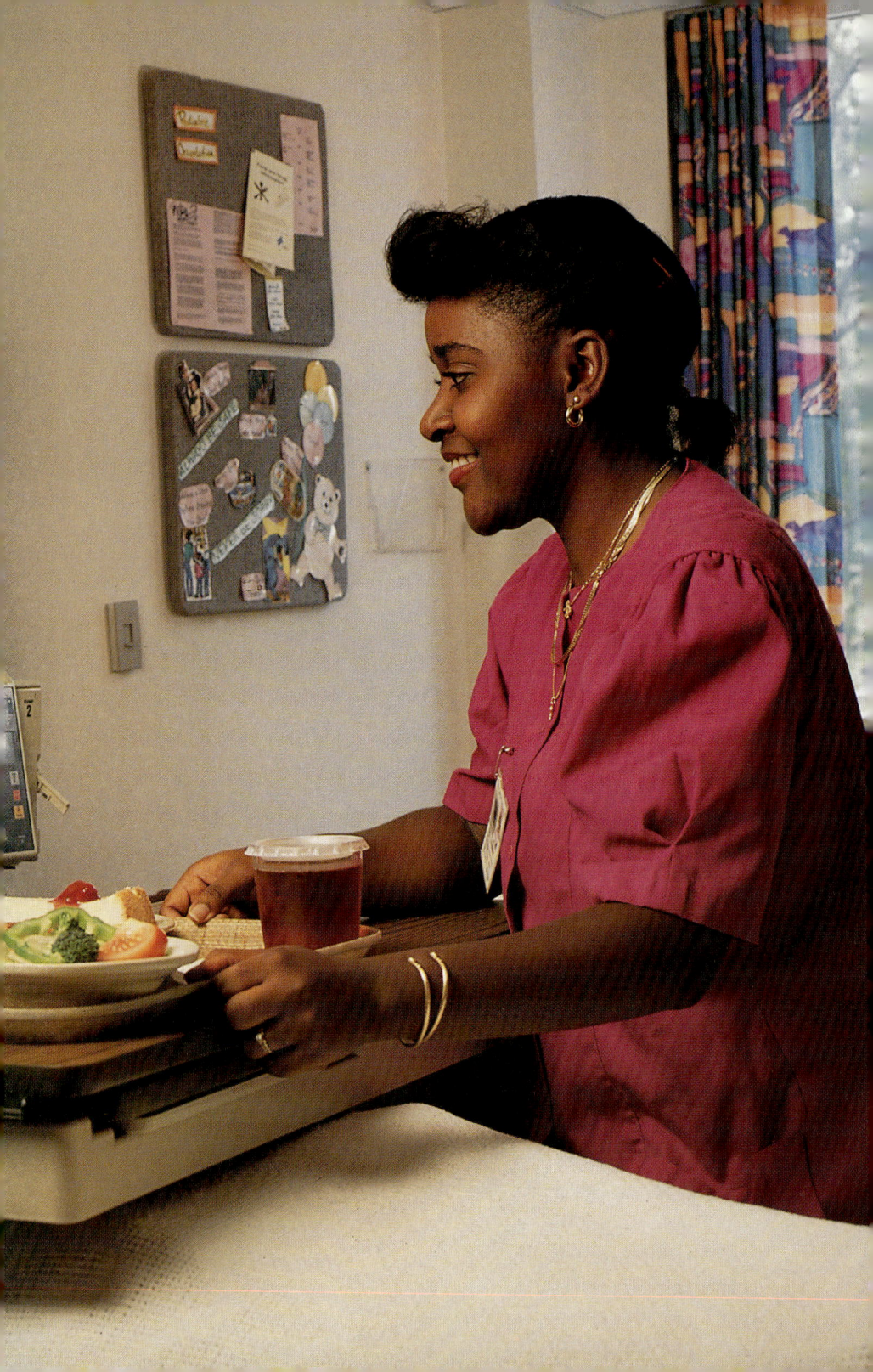

Chapter 5

Where the Job Can Lead

Nurse assistants can advance in several ways. Most advance by gaining experience. Experienced assistants can provide better patient care. They earn higher salaries. Other nurse assistants advance by receiving more training. They usually earn higher salaries if they complete CNA programs.

Most nurse assistants advance by gaining experience.

Some nurse assistants advance by changing job locations. Assistants in nursing homes may advance by taking jobs in hospitals. Assistants who work in small facilities may advance by moving to larger facilities.

Some nurse assistants advance by moving into other health care jobs. Nurse assistants must have extra training to do this. Some assistants become nurses. Most nurses attend two to five years of school after high school. They must earn nursing licenses. Nurses earn salaries much higher than nurse assistants.

Nurse assistant experience prepares people for work as nurses or doctors. Nurse assistants know that they like to work in health care settings. They understand hospital procedures. They know how to maintain patients' files. They understand what it is like to work with patients.

Nurse assistants understand what it is like to work with patients.

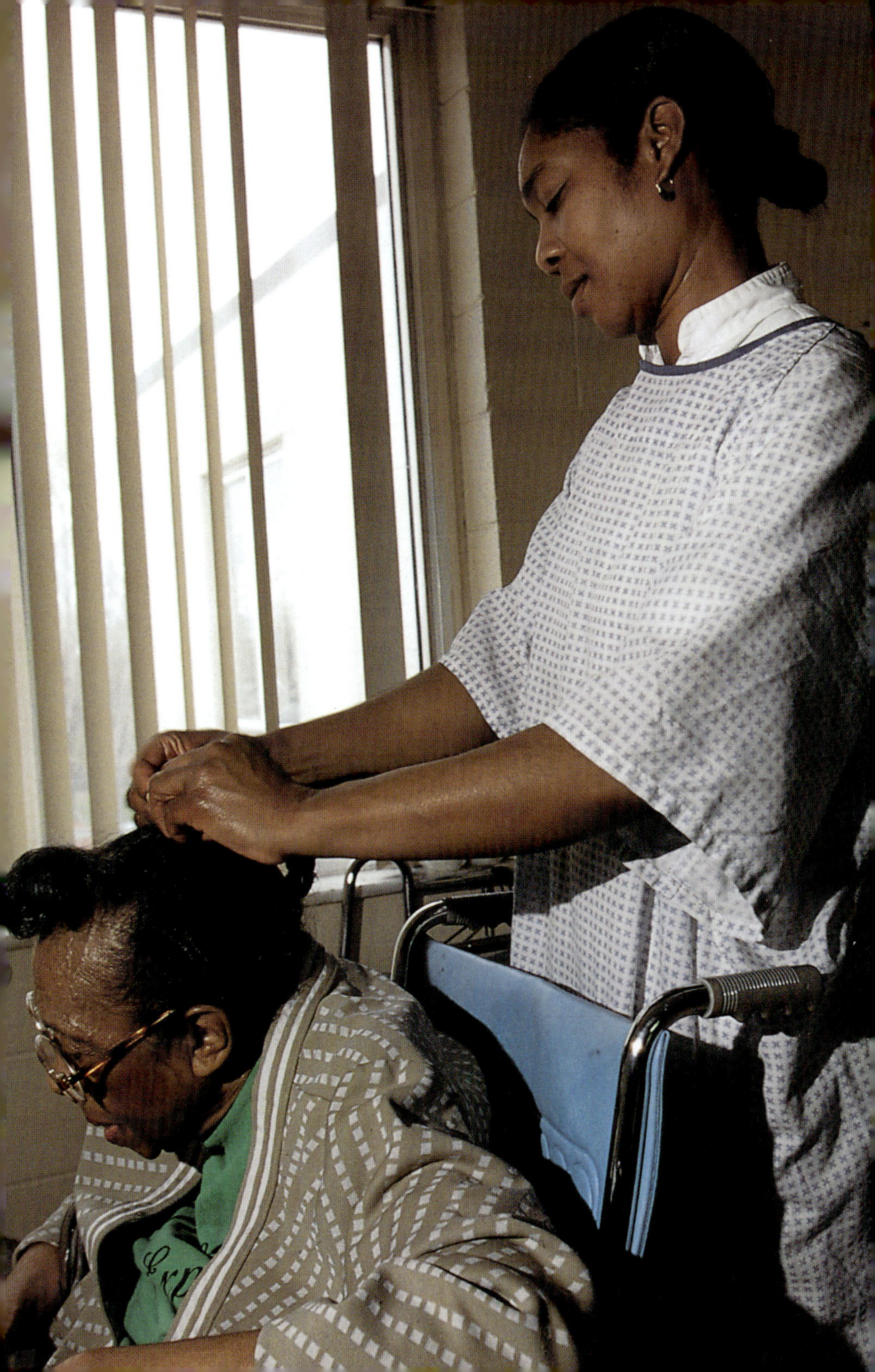

Words to Know

anatomy (uh-NAT-uh-mee)—the study of the body

blood pressure (BLUHD PRESH-ur)—the force blood places on arteries as it moves through the body

certified (SUR-tuh-fide)—having officially recognized training, skills, and abilities

examination (eg-zam-uh-NAY-shuhn)—a careful check of a person's medical condition; nurse assistants take patients to examination rooms.

geriatric (jer-ee-AT-rik)—having to do with older people; nurse assistants who care for older people are geriatric aides.

nutrition (noo-TRISH-uhn)—the study of how bodies use food to stay strong and healthy

procedure (pruh-SEED-jur)—a set way of doing something; nurse assistants follow safety procedures to stay healthy.

pulse (PUHLSS)—the throbbing in the veins caused by the heart as it pumps blood

temperature (TEM-pur-uh-chur)—the measure of how hot or cold something is; nurse assistants check patients' body temperatures.

thermometer (thur-MOM-uh-tur)—a tool that measures temperature

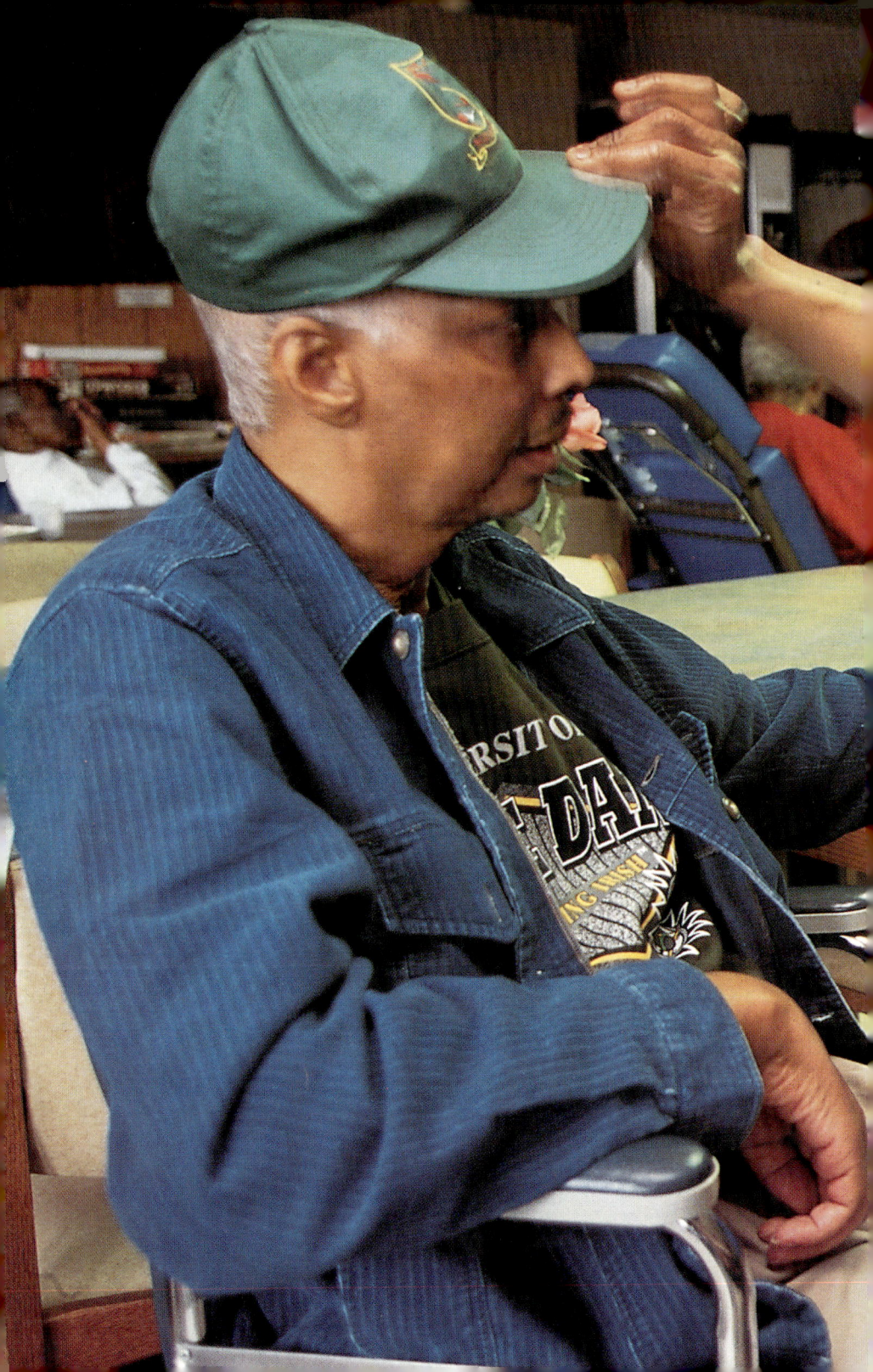

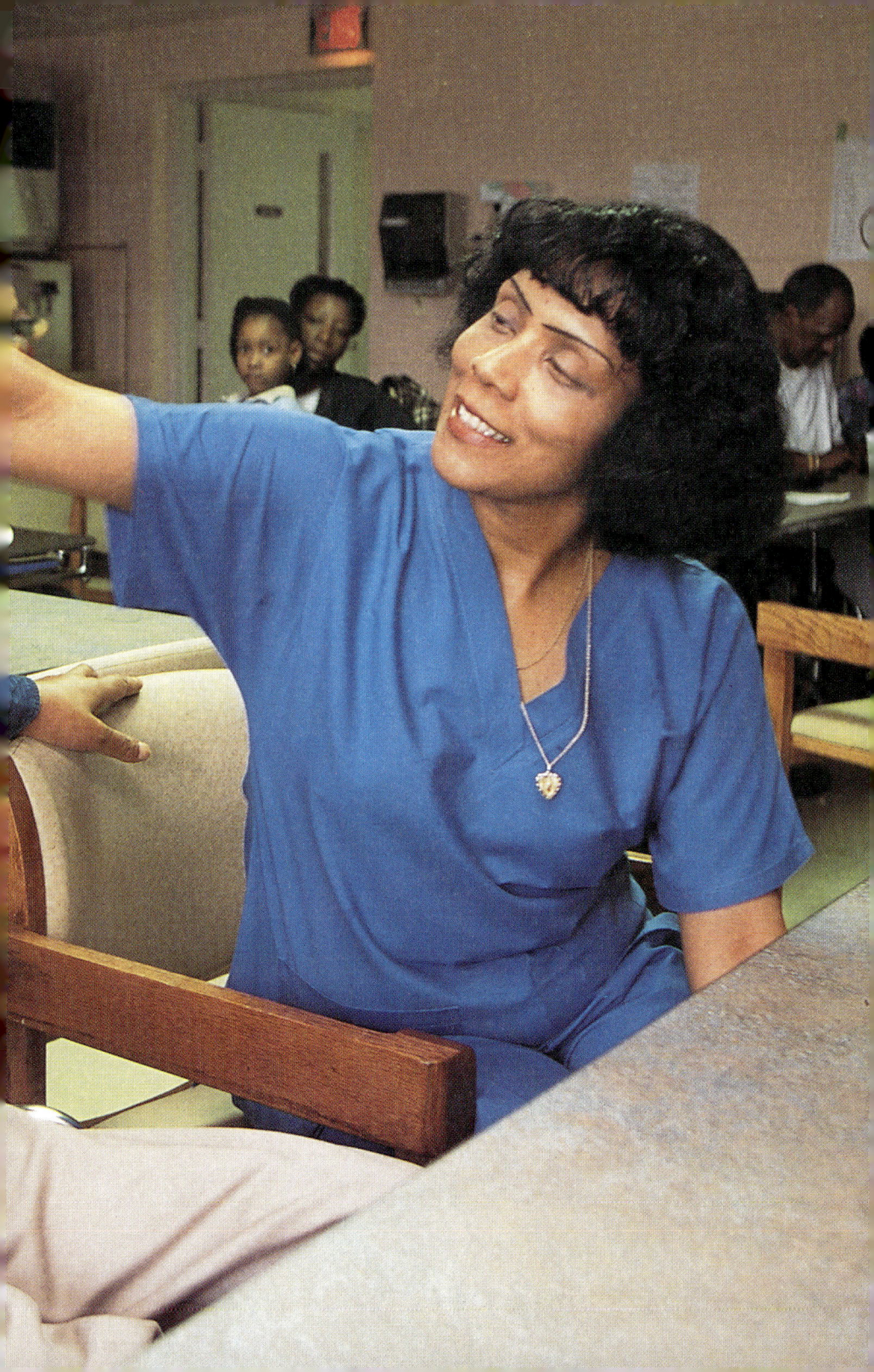

To Learn More

Field, Shelly. *Career Opportunities in Health Care.* New York: Facts on File, 1997.

Lund, Bill. *A Career in Health Care. Getting Ready.* Minneapolis: Capstone Press, 1996.

Simon, Charnan. *Home Health Aide.* Careers without College. Mankato, Minn.: Capstone Press, 1998.

Snook, I. Donald, Jr. *Opportunities in Health and Medical Careers.* Lincolnwood, Ill.: VGM Career Horizons, 1998.

Wilkinson, Beth. *Careers inside the World of Health Care.* New York: Rosen Publishing Group, 1995.

Useful Addresses

Council for Nursing Assistants
LeMarchant Medical Centre
195 LeMarchant Road
St. John's, New Foundland A1C 2H5
Canada

**National Association
  of Geriatric Nursing Assistants**
1706 East Fourth Street
Joplin, MO 64801

National League for Nursing
61 Broadway
New York, NY 10006

Internet Sites

Canada Job Futures
http://www.hrdc-drhc.gc.ca/JobFutures/english/volume1/341/341.htm

Entry-Level Health Care Careers
http://www.workready.org/entrylev.html

National Association of Health Career Schools Online
http://www.nahcs.org/index.html

Occupational Outlook Handbook—Nursing Aides and Psychiatric Aides
http://stats.bls.gov/oco/ocos165.htm

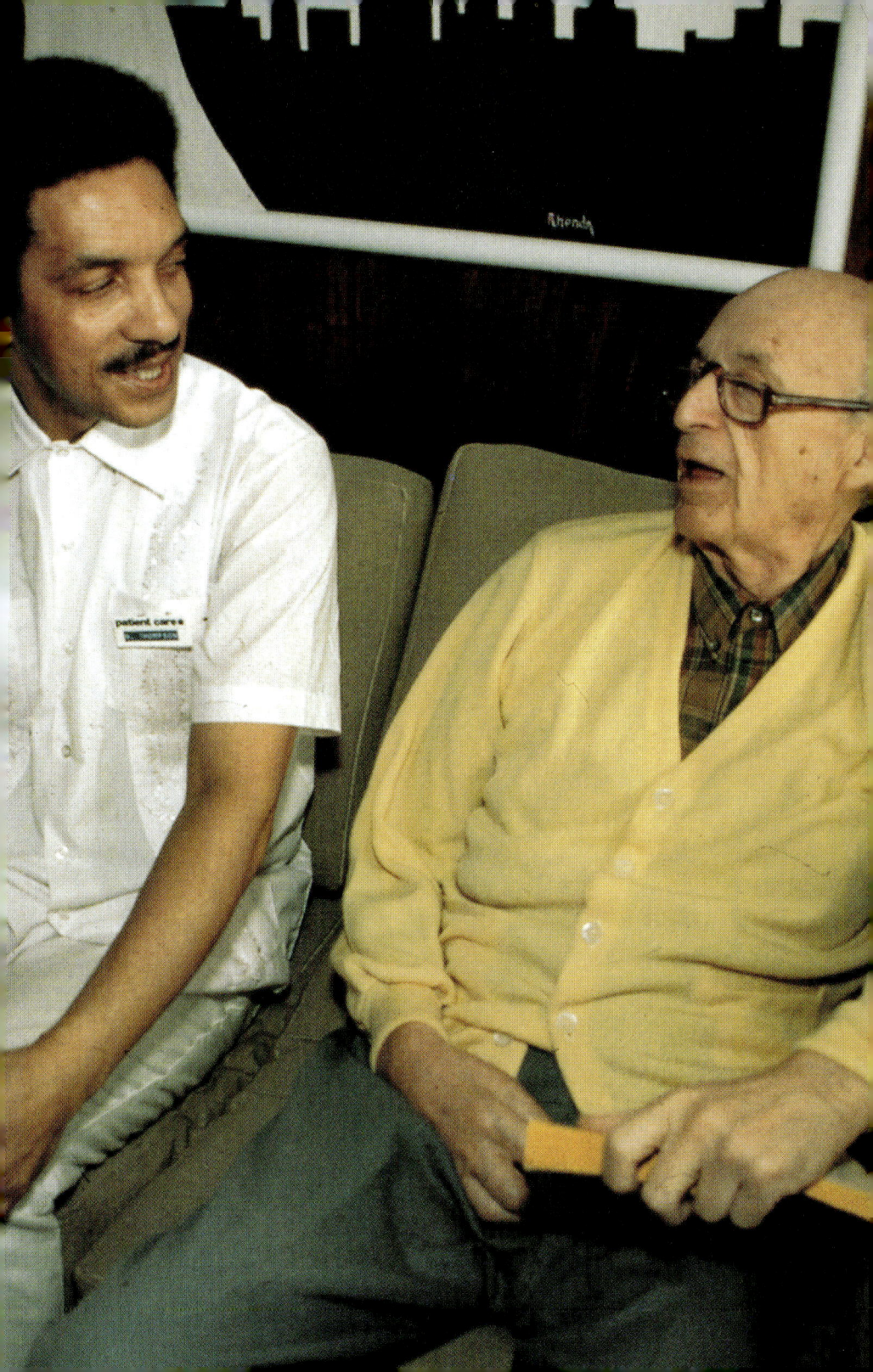

Index

certified nursing assistants (CNAs), 24, 27, 37
class, 24, 27
community college, 23

doctors, 7, 10, 18, 21, 35, 38

files, 38
full-time, 32

geriatric aides, 7

high school, 23, 24, 28, 38
home health aides, 15
hospital, 15, 17, 24, 28, 31, 35, 38
hours, 17

licenses, 24, 38

medical test, 8, 10

nurses, 7, 8, 10, 18, 21, 35, 38
nursing home, 13, 15, 17, 24, 28, 31, 32, 35, 38

part-time, 17

residential care center 5, 15, 32, 35
risks, 18

tasks, 8, 17, 35
test, 8, 10, 27

vocational schools, 23
volunteers, 28